TEEN GUIDE TO MENTAL HEALTH

TEEN GUIDE:
DEPRESSION

by Mary Bates

BrightPoint Press

San Diego, CA

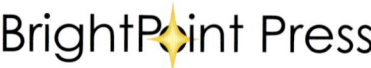

© 2026 BrightPoint Press
an imprint of ReferencePoint Press, Inc.
Printed in the United States

For more information, contact:
BrightPoint Press
PO Box 27779
San Diego, CA 92198
www.BrightPointPress.com

ALL RIGHTS RESERVED.

No part of this work covered by the copyright hereon may be reproduced or used in any form or by any means—graphic, electronic, or mechanical, including photocopying, recording, taping, web distribution, or information storage retrieval systems—without the written permission of the publisher.

Content Consultant: Pardis Khosravi, PsyD, Clinical Director at Children's Health Council and Adjunct Professor at the University of San Francisco

LIBRARY OF CONGRESS CATALOGING-IN-PUBLICATION DATA

Name: Bates, Mary, author.
Title: Teen guide: depression / by Mary Bates.
Description: San Diego, CA: ReferencePoint Press, 2026 | Series: Teen guide to mental health | Audience: Grade 7 to 9 | Includes bibliographical references and index.
Identifiers: ISBN: 9781678211424 (hardcover) | ISBN: 9781678211431 (eBook)
The complete Library of Congress record is available at www.loc.gov.

CONTENTS

CONTENT WARNING: THIS BOOK DESCRIBES SUICIDE AND SUICIDAL THOUGHTS, WHICH MAY BE TRIGGERING TO SOME READERS.

AT A GLANCE	4
INTRODUCTION SAM'S STORY	6
CHAPTER ONE WHAT IS DEPRESSION?	12
CHAPTER TWO THE IMPACTS OF DEPRESSION	28
CHAPTER THREE TREATMENT AND SUPPORT	40
Glossary	58
Source Notes	59
For Further Research	60
Index	62
Image Credits	63
About the Author	64

AT A GLANCE

- Depression is a mood disorder that causes persistent feelings of sadness and hopelessness. It can affect how a person thinks, feels, and behaves.

- Depression is caused by a combination of factors. Some factors are biological while others are environmental.

- Going through puberty can contribute to depression. Teens might face peer pressure, academic expectations, and changing bodies during this time.

- Rates of depression among US teens have increased since the early 2000s. Possible reasons include social media and stressful life events.

- Teen girls, teens who identify as LGBTQ+, and teens who identify as certain races or ethnicities are at a higher risk for depression.

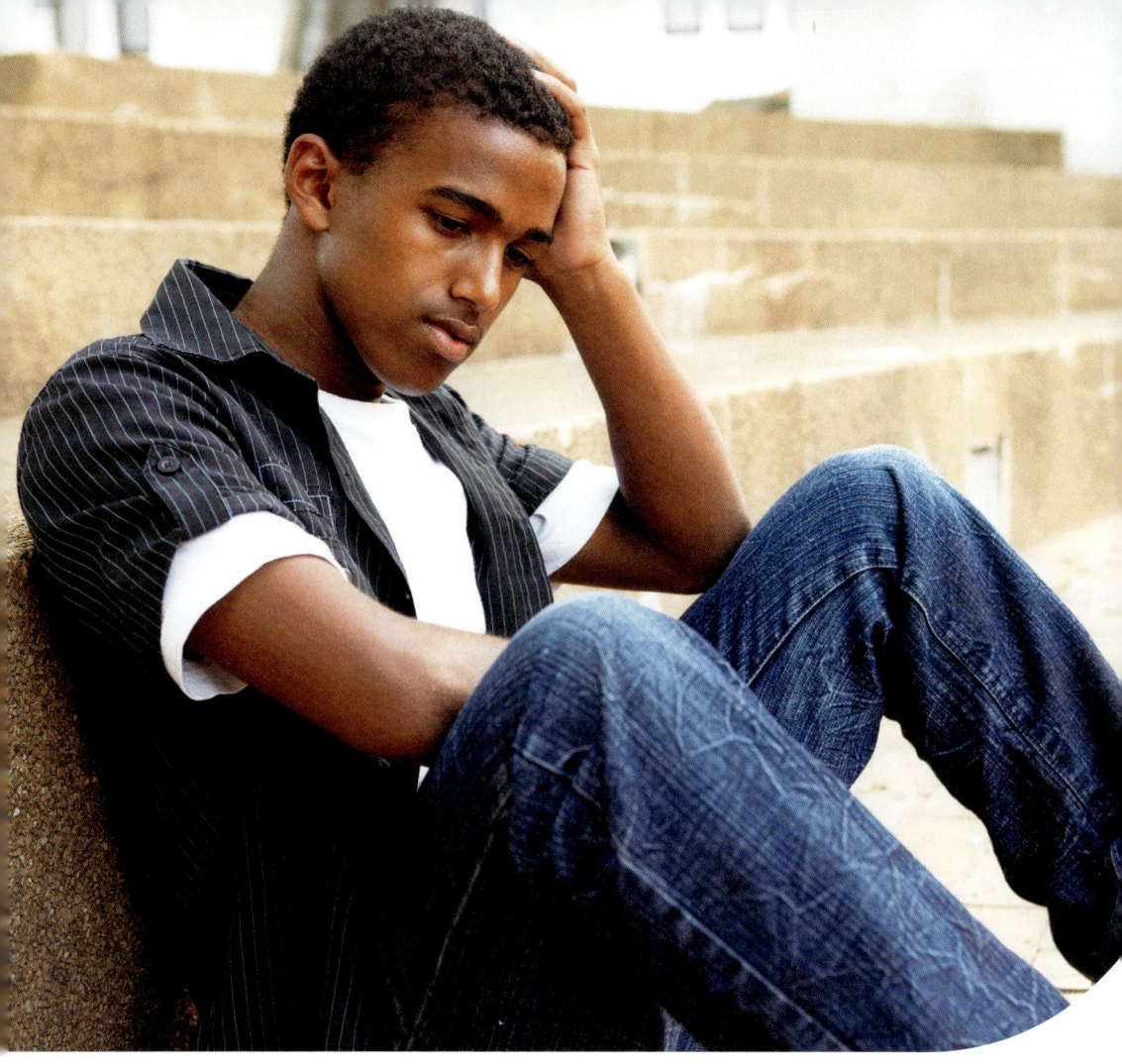

- Teen depression can worsen without treatment and may lead to social or academic problems, substance abuse, self-harm, and suicide.

- Depression can be treated with therapy, medications, or both. With treatment and support, teens can better manage their depression.

INTRODUCTION

SAM'S STORY

Sam's life seemed perfect. She had a supportive family and close friends. She was a good student. And she was a talented athlete. But Sam suffered a sports injury her sophomore year of high school. She could no longer take part in any athletics. Sports gave her a sense of identity and belonging. Sam did not know who she was without them.

Sports injuries can be both physically and mentally challenging for some teens to deal with.

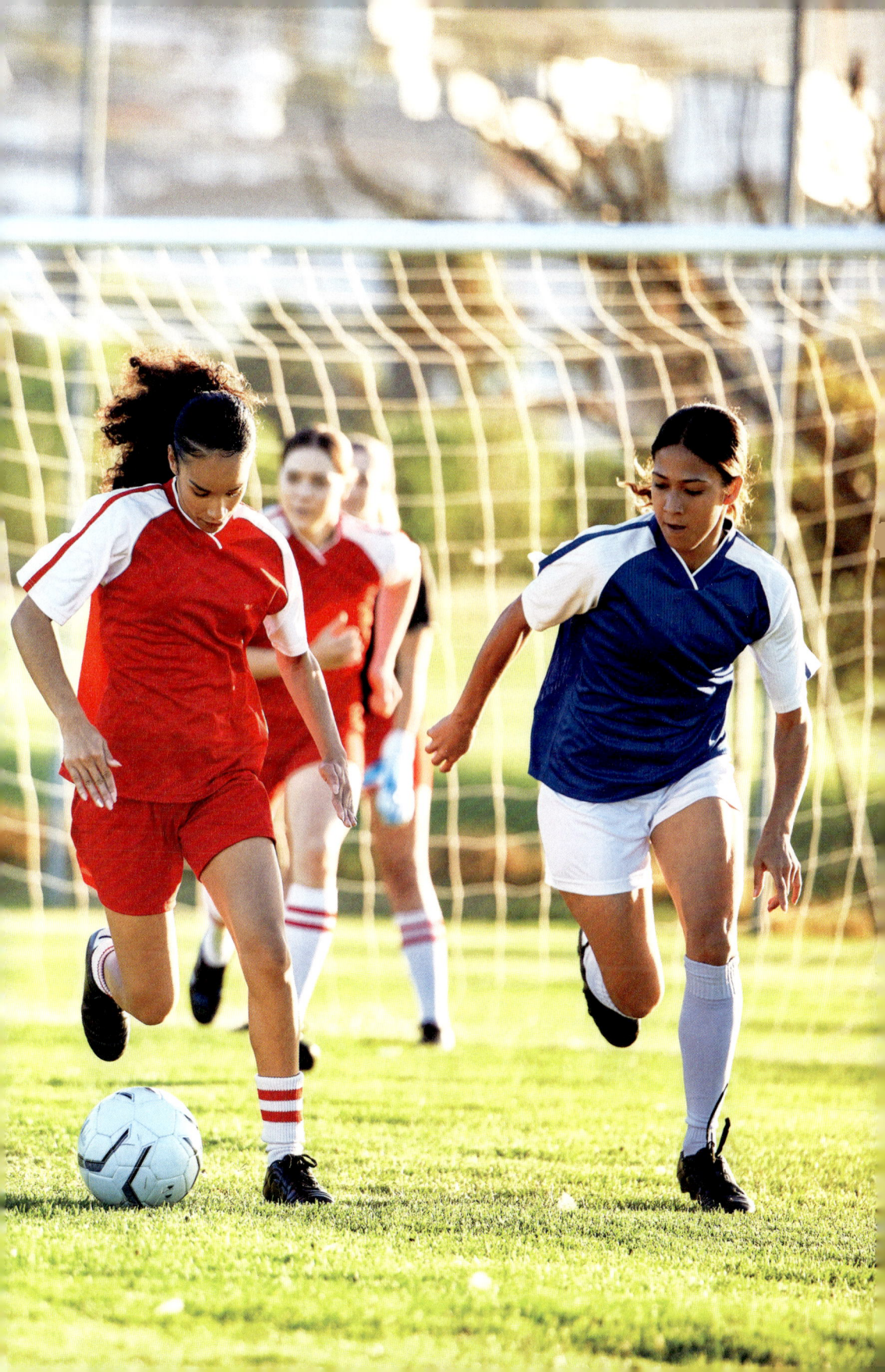

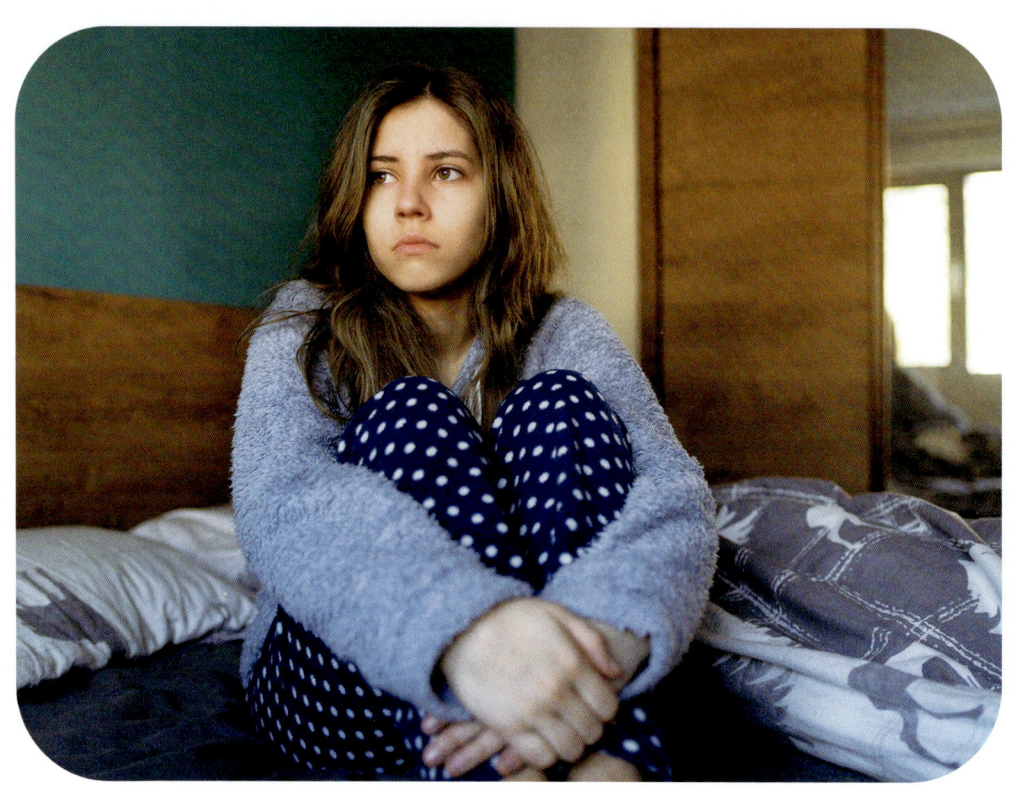

Teens dealing with depression may feel more tired or have less energy than their peers.

Sam started feeling alone. She felt different from her peers. She withdrew from her friends. And Sam often thought about suicide. She did not tell anyone how she felt. Sam began cutting herself to **cope** with her negative feelings. It gave her a temporary sense of control. But after she did it, she felt worse.

Sam knew that cutting was not a healthy way to deal with her problems. She decided to tell her mom about her struggles. Her mom was surprised. But she wanted to get Sam the help she needed.

After speaking to her doctor, Sam was referred to a mental health program.

Many teens have a hard time expressing their mental health struggles with friends and family members.

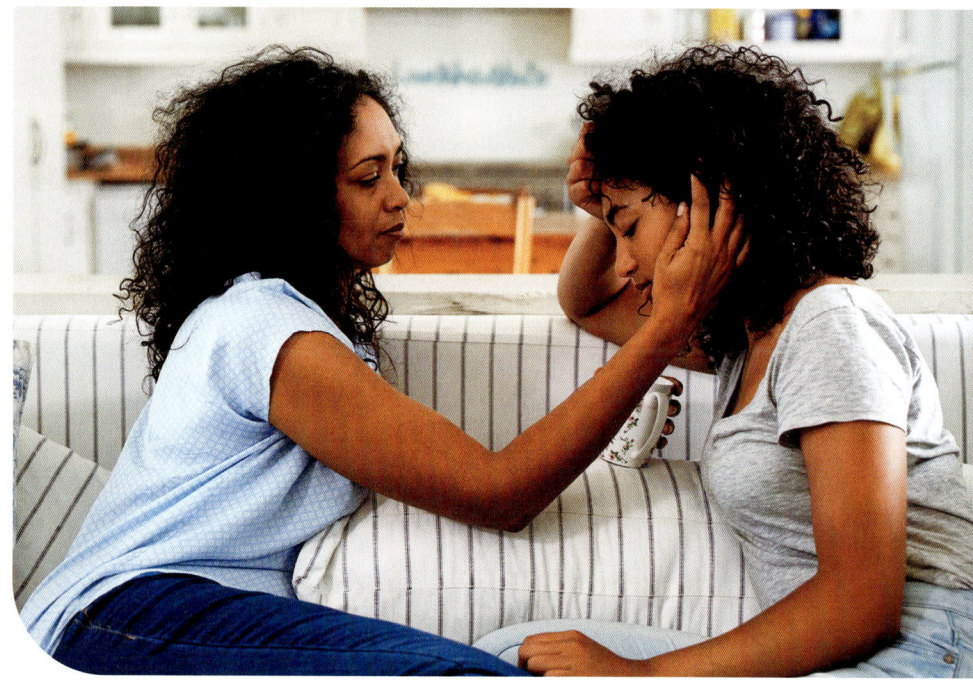

The program helped treat her depression. Sam learned healthier ways to cope with her negative thoughts and feelings. She said, "The staff worked with me and gave me the tools I needed to get better and inspired me to *want* to feel better."[1]

EXPERIENCING DEPRESSION

Like Sam, people with depression are more than just sad. Depression affects people's thoughts, emotions, and physical health. Millions of people around the United States deal with depression. Teens are especially at risk.

Depression can have serious, long-term consequences. But there is help for those who are struggling. Treatment and support can help teens with depression get better.

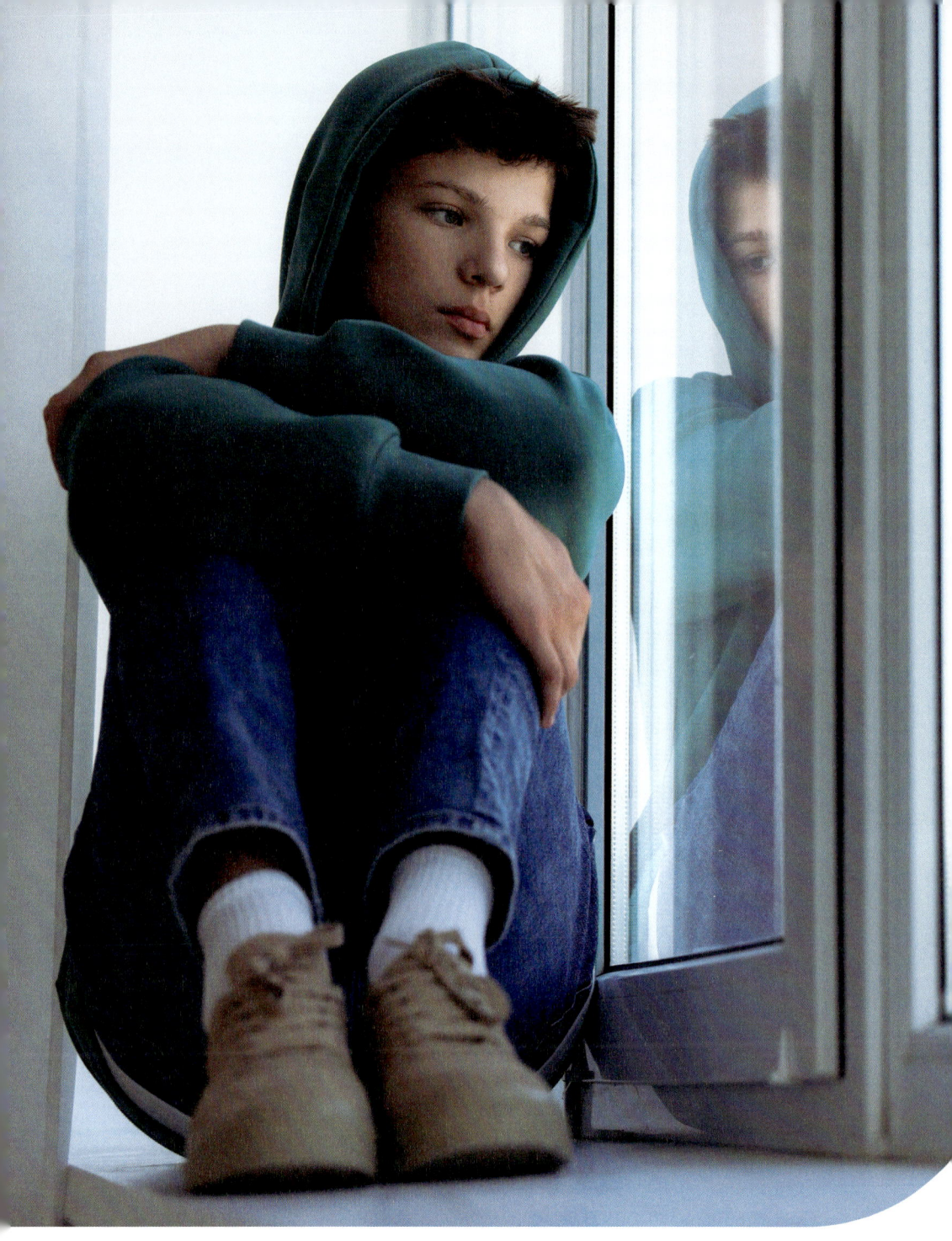

Depression is one of the most common mental health disorders in the United States.

CHAPTER ONE

WHAT IS DEPRESSION?

Major depression is a common mood disorder. It is also known as clinical depression. Depression causes severe feelings of sadness and hopelessness. It can also make people easily annoyed or angered. Depression can affect how a person thinks, feels, and behaves.

People can develop depression at any age. But it often begins in the early teens.

One form of clinical depression is seasonal depression. It occurs during certain seasons of the year, mainly in the fall and winter.

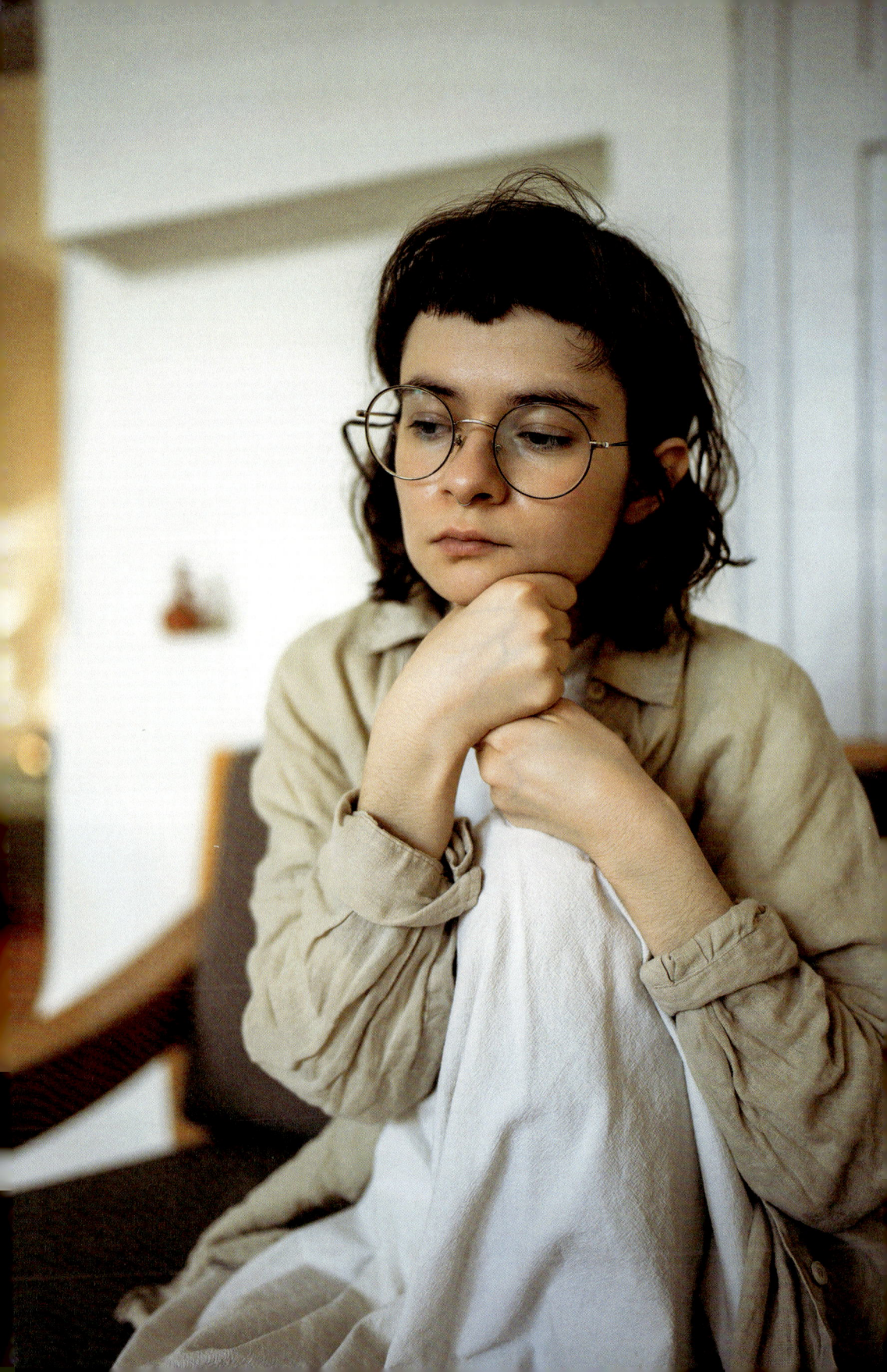

Recognizing the signs of depression in teens may be especially challenging.

Gurinder Dabhia is a pediatrician from San Diego, California. She says it is common for teens to be moody. Dabhia explains, "They're going through physical changes and asking questions about who

Teens dealing with depression might get into more arguments with their parents or caregivers than their peers.

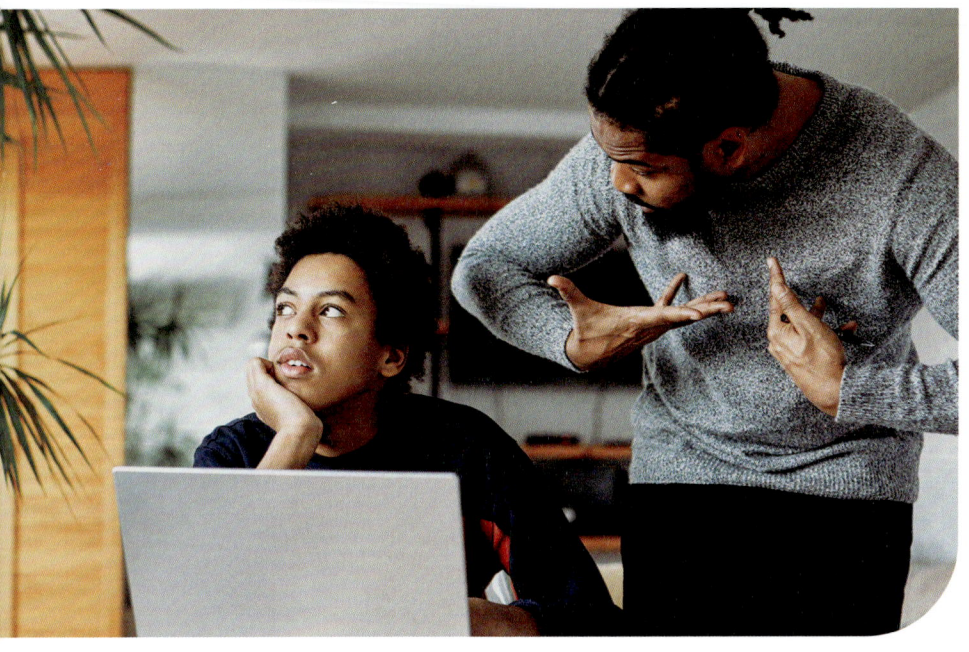

they are and what they want to do with their lives."[2] Dabhia states that occasional bad moods and acting out can be normal. But extreme changes in mood and behavior can be a sign of depression.

SIGNS AND SYMPTOMS

Not everyone with depression has the same symptoms. A person must have several symptoms for at least two weeks to be **diagnosed**. These symptoms must be serious enough to cause problems in a person's daily life. Symptoms may include changes in emotions, thoughts, and behaviors.

Changes in mood are a common sign of depression. People with depression often feel sad, hopeless, or easily angered.

They may feel worthless or guilty. They may also have low **self-esteem**. Depression can make teens stop enjoying activities they once did. These include hobbies or spending time with friends.

Depression can affect the way people think. It can make it hard to focus, make decisions, or remember things. People with depression may feel negatively about their life and the future. They may have frequent thoughts about death or suicide.

Another sign of depression is sensitivity to rejection or failure. People with depression may be hard on themselves. This was the case for Avary Whitehead. In 2024, the 16-year-old talked about his experience with depression. He said, "I [would] always look back and think

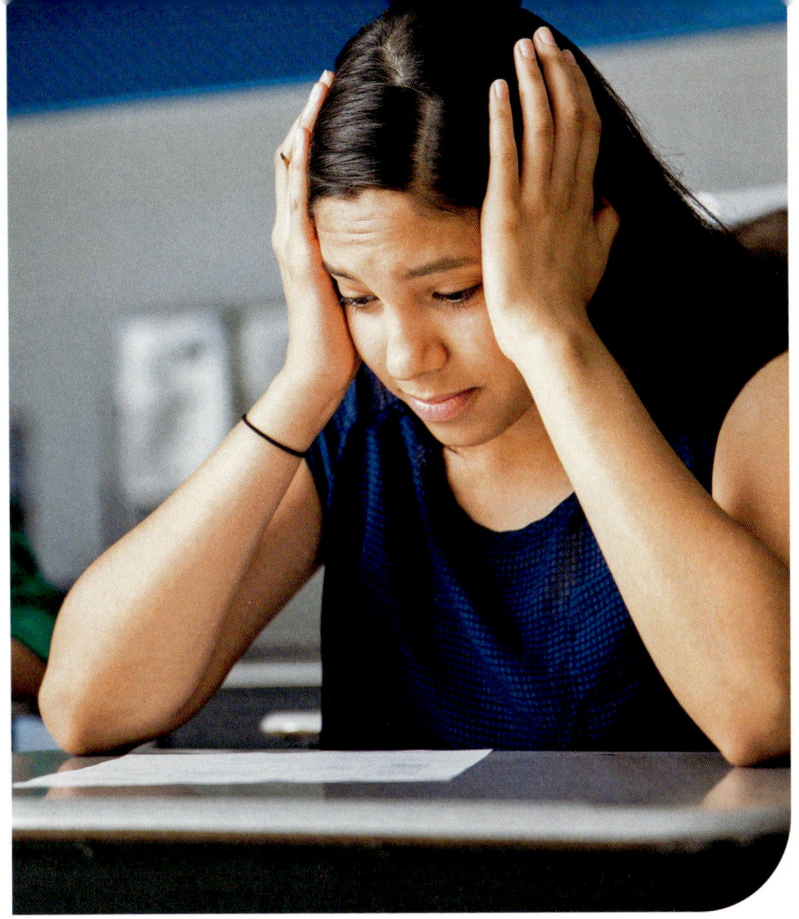

Constant stress is harmful to teens and can increase their chances for developing depression.

negatively about myself or about the actions or decisions I made."[3]

Depression can cause people to act differently than usual. People with depression may isolate themselves. They may seem angrier. They may take part in risky or harmful behaviors. These include abusing drugs or alcohol, self-harming, and attempting suicide.

Some people have physical symptoms of depression. For example, people may have changes in their appetite or eating habits. Their sleeping habits might also change. They may feel more tired. They could have low energy. Or they can feel restless and agitated. Depression can also cause frequent headaches or stomachaches.

HOW COMMON IS TEEN DEPRESSION?

Depression among teens rose during the 2000s. In the United States, the rate of teen depression almost doubled between 2009 and 2019. Experts continue to research the reasons for this increase.

One factor may be the rise in technology use. In the early 2010s, teens started spending more time on social media. This caused some teens to feel lonelier. Technology may contribute to depression in a few ways. For example, it may cause teens to spend less time with others in person. Research shows that in-person socializing is good for one's mental health.

Social Media and Mental Health

About 95 percent of teens use social media. One-third say they use social media almost all the time. Social media can have benefits. But it also presents risks. Spending more than three hours a day on social media can make teens twice as likely to have mental health problems. These include developing depression.

Social media may also affect mental health. Some teens may compare themselves to others online. They might compare their body type or interests. This can cause some teens to feel different from their peers.

Other factors also contribute to teen depression. Teens today face many global stresses. These include climate change, gun violence, and economic struggles. Issues such as those may make teens feel uncertain about the future.

Kathleen Ethier works at the Centers for Disease Control and Prevention. She says, "We've known for a while that mental health among young people was going in the wrong direction."[4] Experts have known about teens' mental health struggles for years. But the problem grew in 2020. This was due to the COVID-19 pandemic.

The pandemic affected people in different ways. Most teens faced social isolation. They also dealt with disruptions in their schooling. Many also lost a loved

During the COVID-19 pandemic, many students had to take virtual classes rather than learning in a classroom alongside their peers.

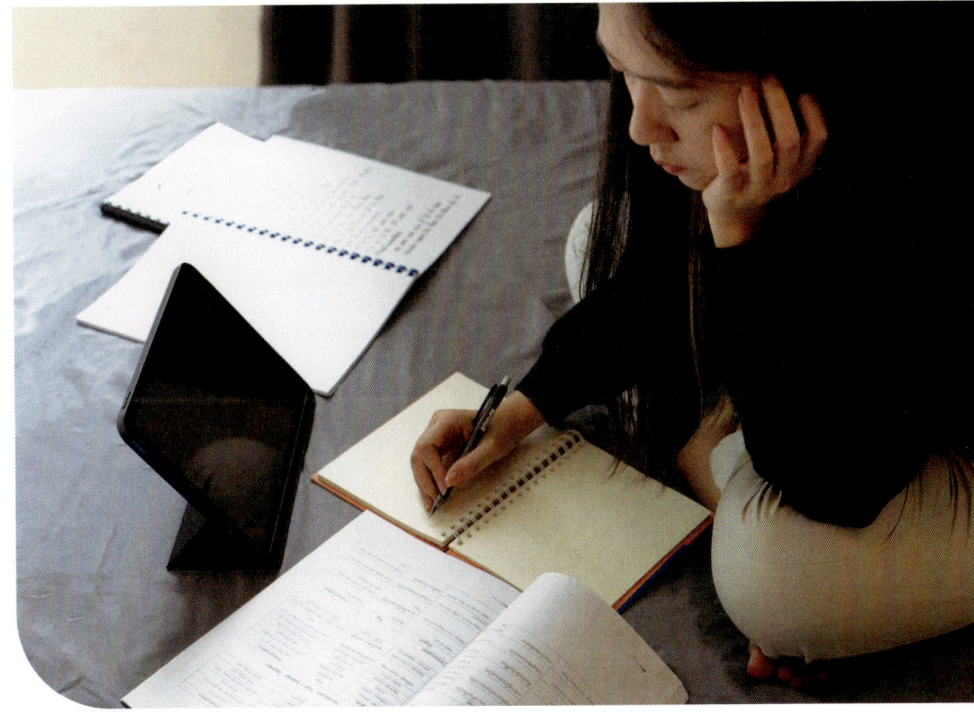

one to COVID-19. Some had parents lose their jobs. These stresses may have greatly affected teen mental health. In 2021, about 20 percent of US teens had symptoms of major depression. That was up from about 16 percent in 2019.

Depression also affects some groups more than others. Teen girls have higher rates of depression than teen boys. In 2021, about 30 percent of girls between 12 and 17 years old experienced depression. That was more than twice the number of teen boys who had depression. Teens in the LGBTQ+ community are more at risk for depression. Certain racial and ethnic groups are at risk as well. Depression rates are high for American Indian and Native Alaskan teens.

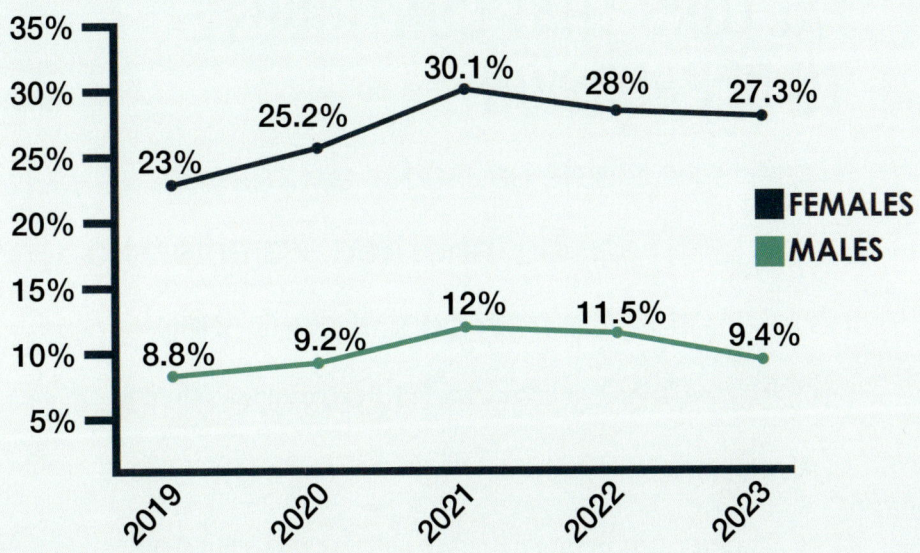

Source: Preeti Vankar, "Percentage of US Youths with a Major Depressive Episode in the Past Year from 2004 to 2023, by Gender," Statista, November 4, 2024. www.statista.com.

A study of about 70,000 teens ages 12 to 17 showed the percentage of those who reported having a major depressive episode between 2019 and 2023.

Teen depression rates have decreased slightly since 2021. But experts are still concerned. The percentage of teens with depression is still much higher than it was in the early 2000s.

FACTORS THAT CONTRIBUTE TO DEPRESSION

There is no single cause for depression. Depression can be **inherited**. Parents who have depression may pass it on to their children. Other close family members may suffer from it too.

Certain situations can also contribute to depression. Stressful life events can increase a person's risk. This could be the death of a loved one. Or it may be family financial struggles. Trauma and abuse can lead to depression as well. So can being a victim of or witness to violence.

Depression can also result from discrimination. Discrimination is when people are treated negatively based on their race, ethnicity, sexual orientation, or gender.

Experts have found a strong link between experiencing racism and developing depression. Racism can take on many forms. These include physical violence and bullying. Those experiences may increase the risk of depression in teens who identify as persons of color.

Bullying can be both physical and verbal, and it can happen in person or online.

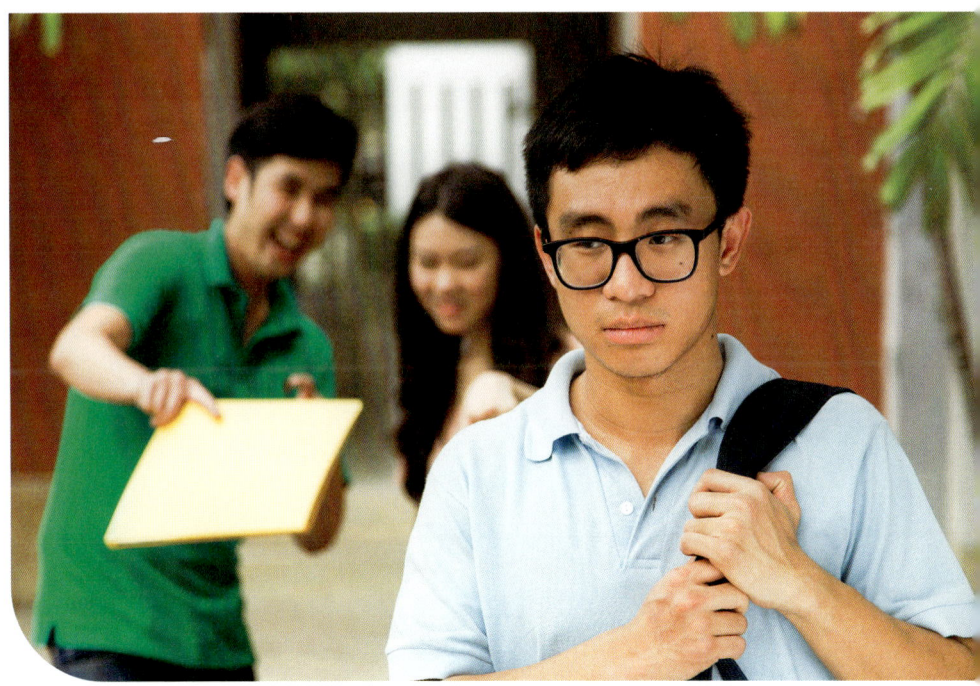

LGBTQ+ teens are at higher risk for depression too. This is especially true if they feel unsupported. In 2023, about 30 percent of LGBTQ+ students were bullied at school. And about 20 percent attempted suicide that year.

Depression rates tend to increase during puberty. Changes in hormones during that time may contribute. Puberty is also a time

Some teens with depression also struggle with eating disorders.

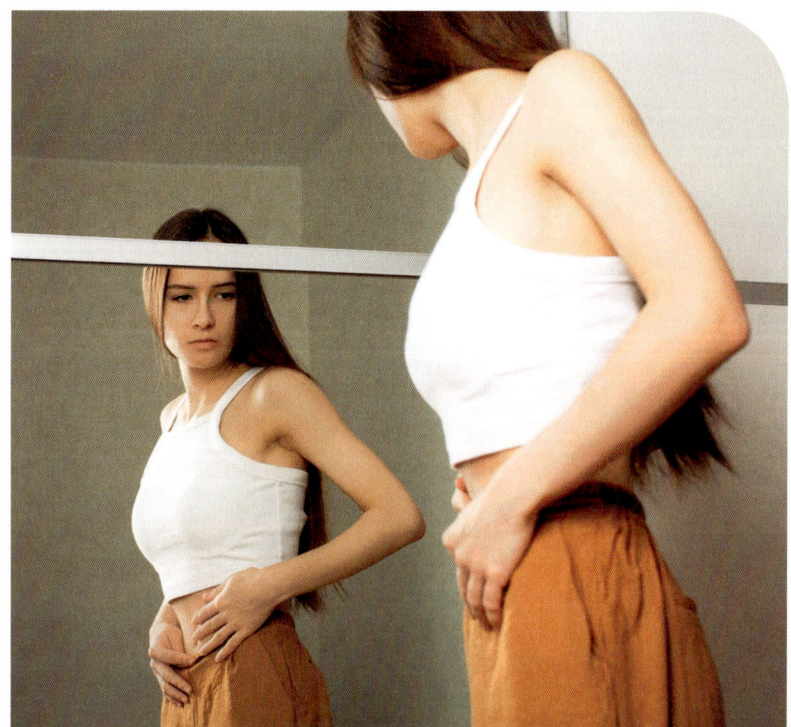

when social relationships change. Teens may deal with new pressures. They may struggle with school. They can also have trouble fitting in socially. Many teens face daily challenges. These challenges may contribute to depression.

Teens with other mental health problems are also at risk for developing depression. These include substance abuse disorder, post-traumatic stress disorder, and anxiety disorders. Learning disabilities and attention-deficit/hyperactivity disorder (ADHD) are also linked to depression. So is having a **chronic** illness.

There are a variety of factors that make depression more likely. But anyone can experience it. Depression affects many teens today. It can have lasting effects.

CHAPTER TWO

THE IMPACTS OF DEPRESSION

Major depression can last for long periods of time. This is especially true when it is left untreated. Depression can go on for weeks, months, or even years. It can affect every part of a teen's life.

Depression may lead to problems at school. It can cause teens to miss school. Teens with depression might have trouble focusing. They might also lose interest in schoolwork. Their grades can go down.

Depression can make it hard for some people to find the motivation to do daily tasks, such as getting out of bed.

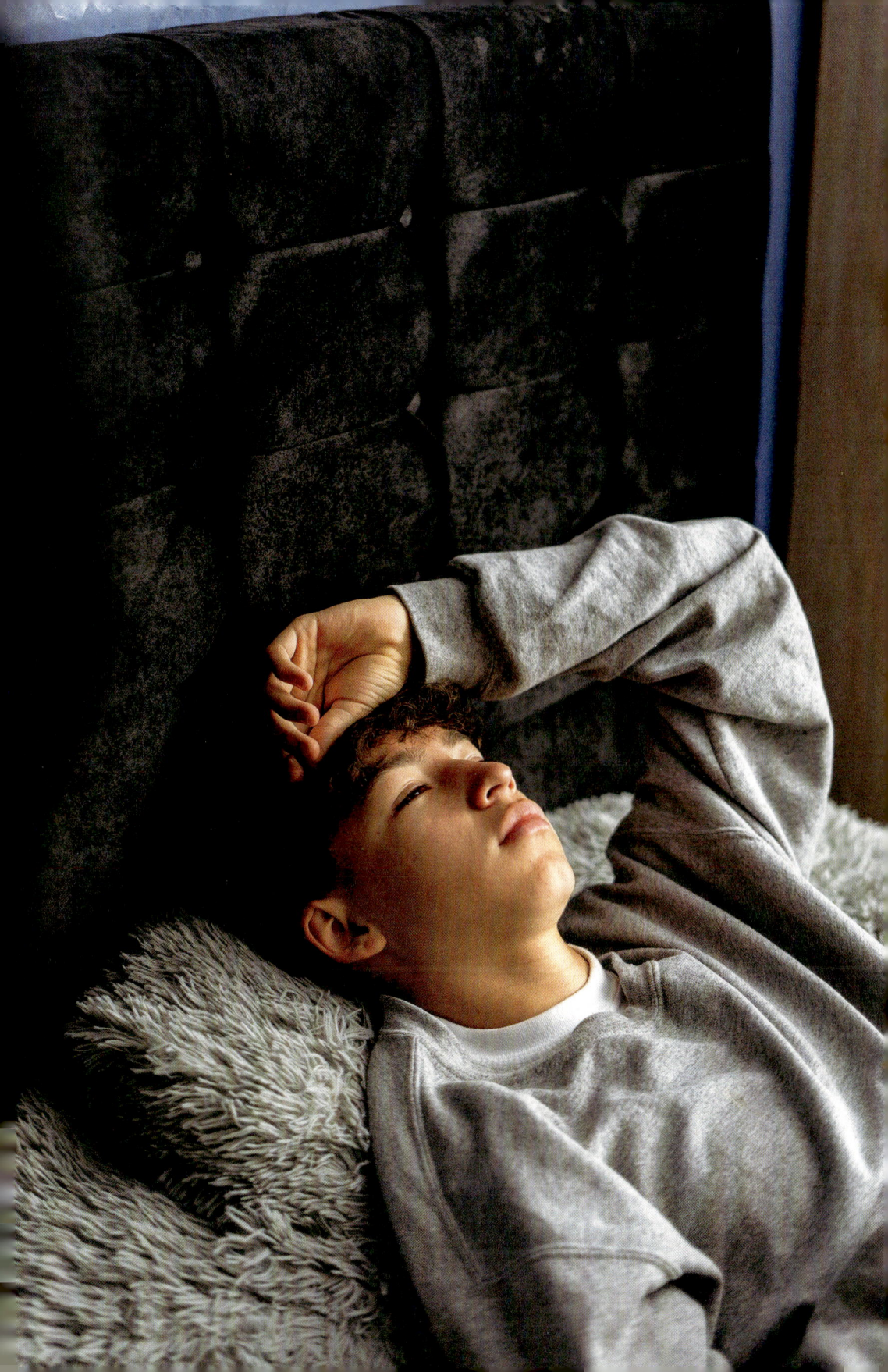

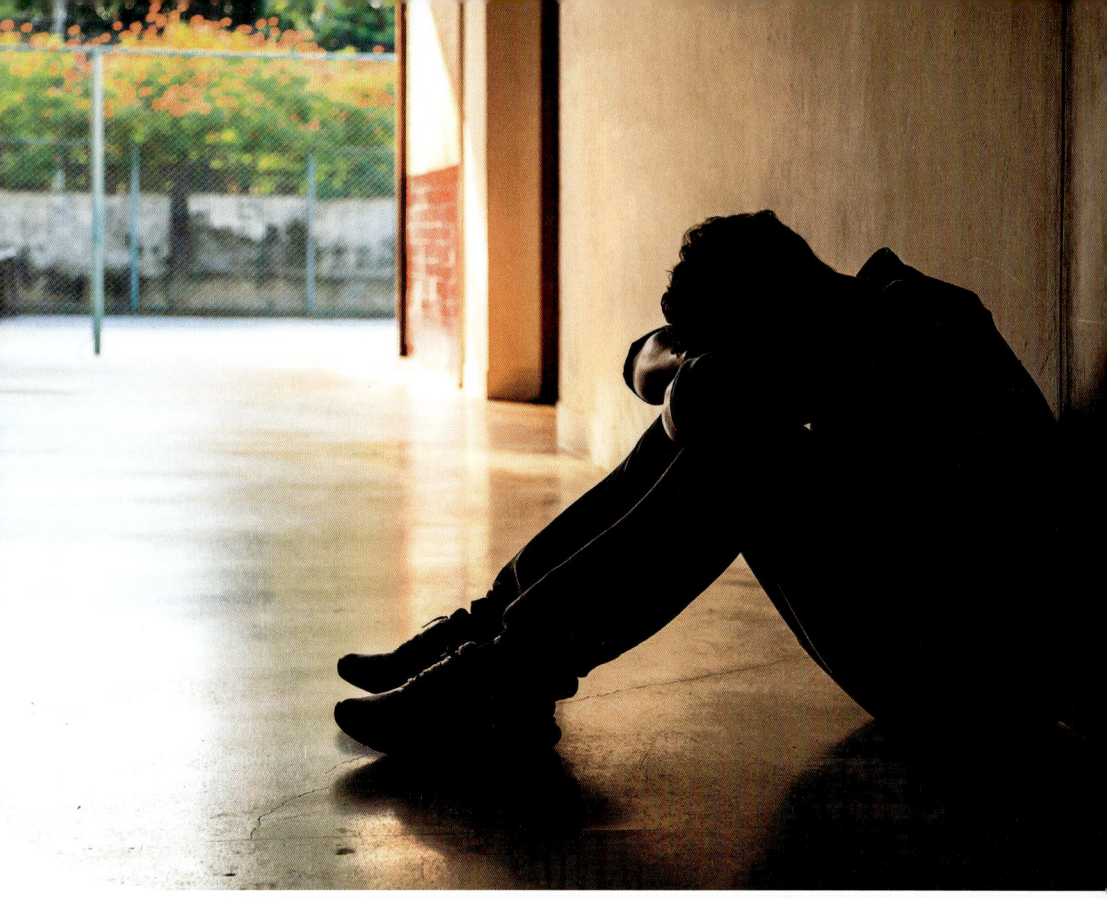

Some teens with depression may refuse to go to school. This can be due to social anxiety, bullying, or academic stress.

Teens with depression may withdraw from their friends. And they may stop doing activities they once enjoyed. These include sports and hobbies.

Morgan is from New Jersey. Her depression made her hate going to school. She said, "I was . . . having issues with my friendships at school and an increased level of stress when it came time for tests, projects, and other assessments."[5]

Social problems are common for teens with depression. They may get into more fights with their family and friends. Depression can cause some teens to feel alone. They might also feel misunderstood. They may even pull away from relationships.

Depression can also cause overwhelming negative emotions. Teens with depression are more likely to use substances to cope with these feelings. These include drugs and alcohol. A 2024 study showed that about 17 percent of teens with depression used drugs or alcohol.

Substance abuse can worsen depression symptoms. It can also cause addiction.

These things can be difficult to overcome. Teens with depression and substance issues face other risks. They are more likely to get arrested by age 19. And they are less likely to finish high school.

Substance abuse can lead to long-term health issues for teens.

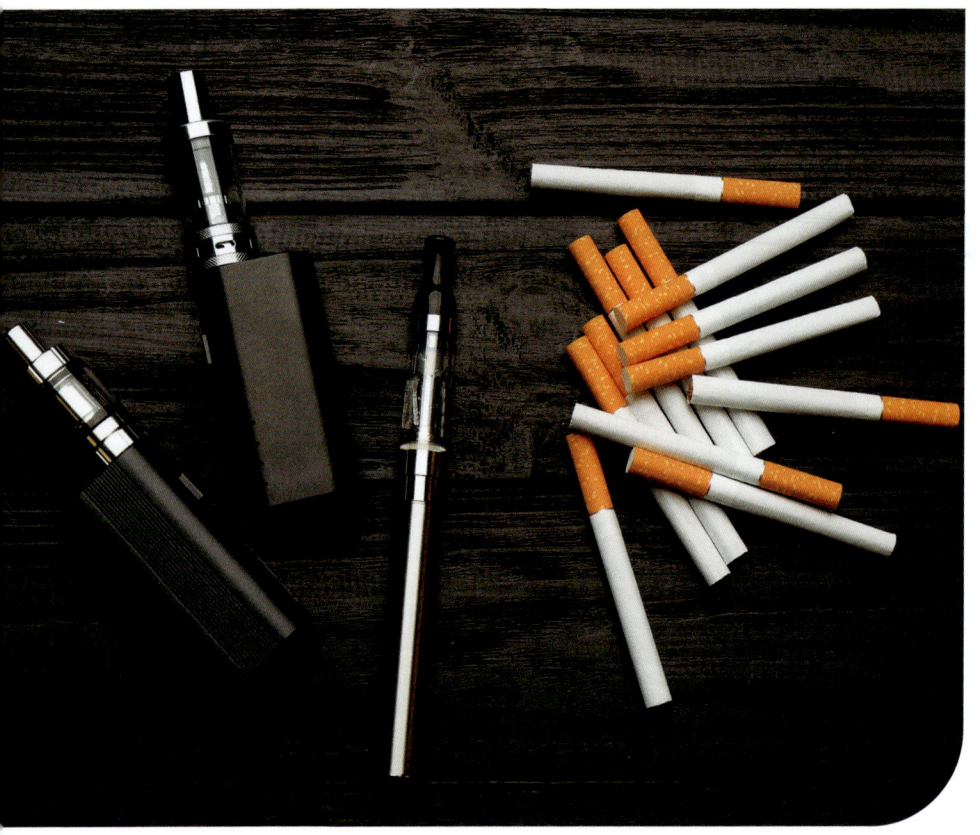

DEPRESSION AND SELF-HARM

Some teens with depression may hurt themselves on purpose. This is known as self-harm. People who self-harm may cut, burn, scratch, or hit themselves. More than half of teens with depression have a history of self-harm.

Teens who self-harm often have trouble coping with their emotions. They may physically hurt themselves to try to deal with their emotional pain. Depression can sometimes make a person feel numb or empty inside. Teens with depression may self-harm to try to feel something. They might also do it to feel a sense of control.

People who self-harm may get short-term relief from their negative emotions. But they

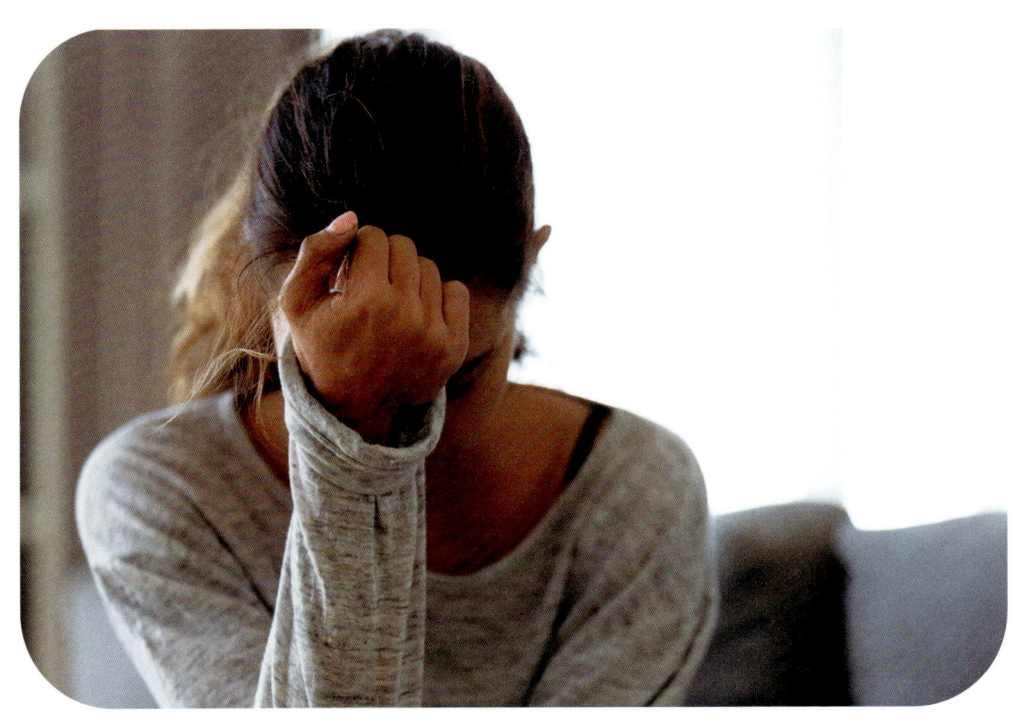

The average age for youths to start self-harming is around 13 years old.

often feel more sadness and guilt later on. This can make negative emotions worsen.

Life issues may increase the risk of self-harm. Teens with family problems or issues at school are more likely to self-harm. Personal trauma also increases the risk. So does having friends who self-harm.

People who self-harm are not attempting suicide. They often hide their injuries.

They do not want others to know what they are doing. Those who self-harm may not want others to know how much they are struggling. However, teens who self-harm have a greater risk of attempting suicide. More than half of children and teens who die by suicide have a history of self-harm.

DEPRESSION AND SUICIDE

Suicide and suicide attempts are often associated with depression. Suicide is a leading cause of death for teens and young adults. In 2023, 22 percent of high school students said they seriously considered suicide in the past year. Many teens who attempt suicide want to end their negative feelings. They think suicide is their only option.

Suicide rates are higher for some groups. Females tend to attempt suicide more often than males. American Indian and Native Alaskan peoples are at increased risk for suicide. Suicide rates are also rising for Black teens. And rates are highest for LGBTQ+ teens.

Jordan Burnham survived a suicide attempt. He attempted suicide his senior year of high school. He talked about his struggle with depression. "I think I was desperate more than anything," he said. "It was hard to find hope, or to see hope."[6]

Burnham shared his story with teens dealing with mental illnesses. He wanted others to understand that they are not alone. He said, "I promise tomorrow, and each day after, will get a little better."[7]

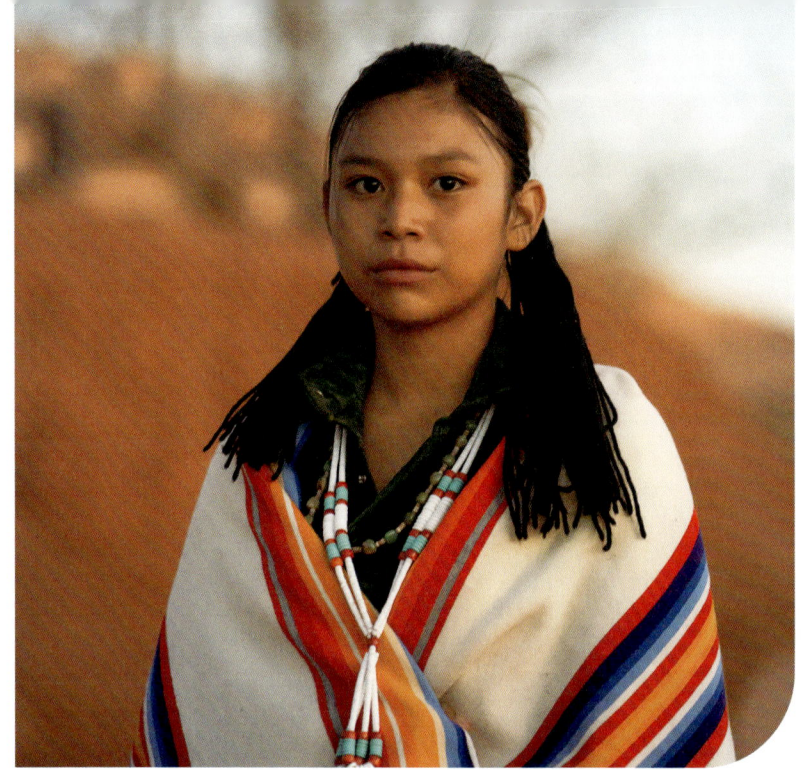

Suicide is the second leading cause of death for American Indian people between 10 and 24 years old.

There are many warning signs that someone may be at risk of suicide. Some signs may not be obvious. People may start giving away important belongings. They might withdraw from friends and family. Other signs are more serious. People who are suicidal may take risks. Those risks could lead to serious injury or death. Some people might share feelings

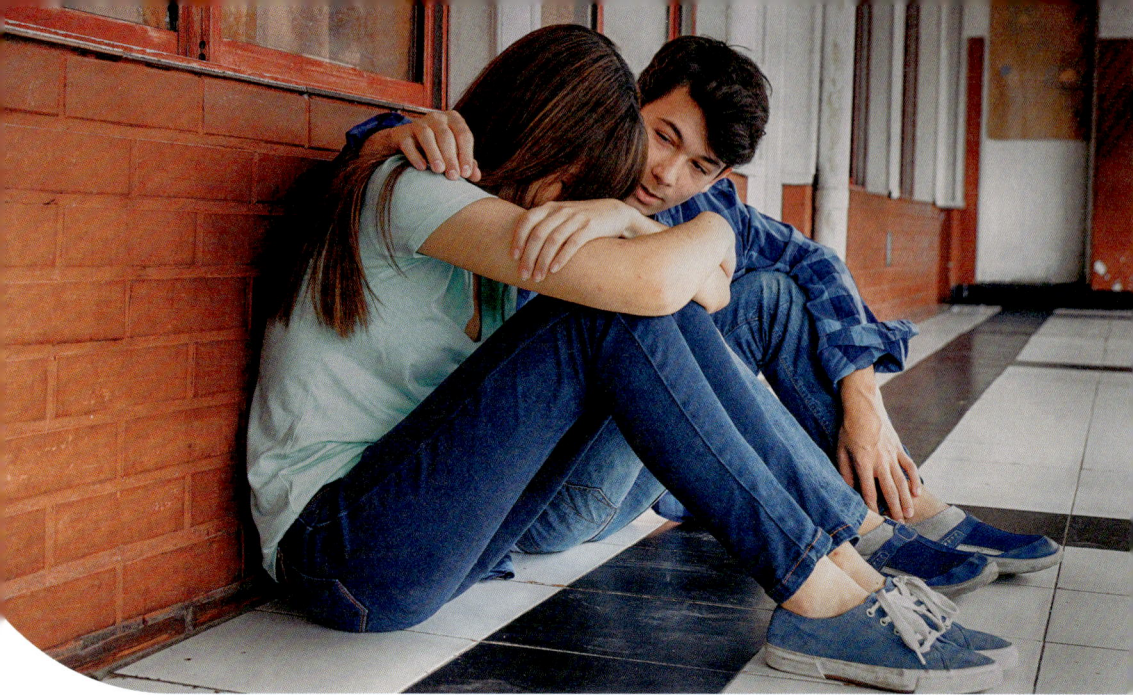

People should not blame or judge someone who is dealing with mental health problems.

of hopelessness. They may even talk about wanting to die or kill themselves.

Any talk or thoughts about suicide should be taken seriously. People should never ignore warning signs of suicide. They should take immediate action if someone is at risk. This may mean talking to the person in a non-judgmental way. It could be checking in on them. It could also be just hanging out with them. Talking to a trusted adult is another option. This could be a parent, teacher, or counselor. Teens can also call a crisis hotline. Emergency services should be called right away if a person attempts suicide.

Symptoms of depression usually do not go away on their own. But many resources are available for those who are struggling. With help and support, teens can overcome depression.

988 Lifeline

People struggling with their mental health can call, text, or chat 988. This is the number for the US suicide and crisis lifeline. The service is available 24 hours every day. It is free to use. People can talk to trained counselors. Counselors provide mental health resources. Those worried about a loved one can use the lifeline too.

CHAPTER THREE

TREATMENT AND SUPPORT

Depression is a treatable mental illness. Teens with depression need different levels of support and treatment. One step to getting treatment is talking with a health-care provider. This could be a family doctor, school nurse, or school counselor. They can refer teens to a mental health professional. These professionals evaluate the person with depression. Then they create a treatment plan.

Men are less likely to seek help for their depression than women.

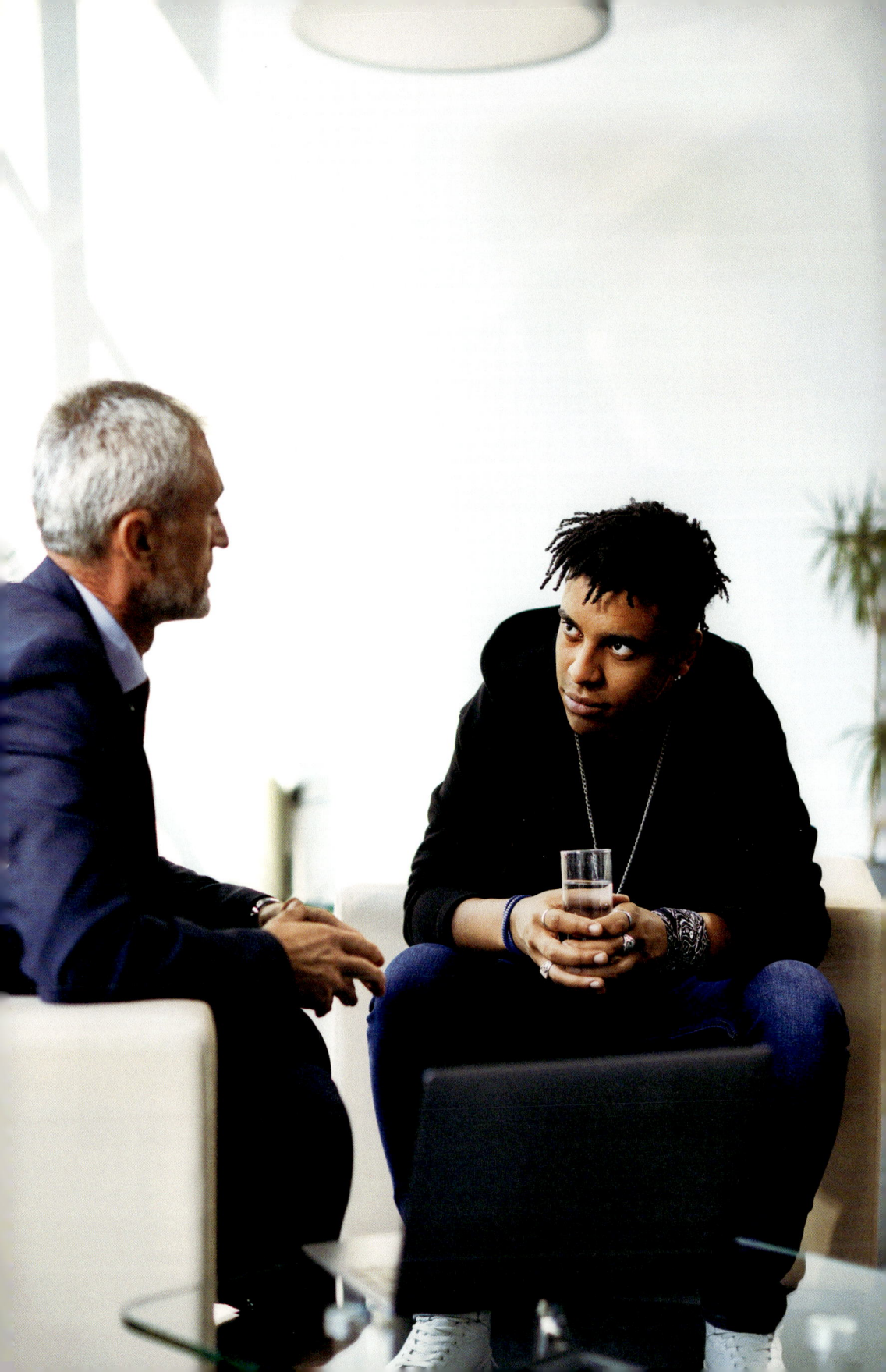

Treatment for depression varies from person to person. It depends on the type and severity of symptoms. Many teens with depression benefit from some form of mental health treatment. One treatment is psychotherapy. This involves talking with a professional mental health provider. Medication can also help.

Access to Treatment

Less than half of teens who need treatment for depression receive it. Accessing treatment can be challenging for many teens. There are several reasons they may not receive mental health treatment. Cost may be one reason. Another is a lack of providers. And some teens may not know how to get help.

In the early 2020s, US teenagers were surveyed about their mental health. About 20 percent said they had received mental health therapy in the past year. And about 14 percent said they took prescription medications for their mental health.

THERAPY

Psychotherapy is also called talk therapy or psychological counseling. It can help teens understand and deal with negative thoughts and feelings. Therapy may help people understand the causes of their depression. Mental health professionals can help teens identify unhealthy behaviors. They help teens find ways to change those behaviors. Therapy is a place to learn coping and problem-solving skills.

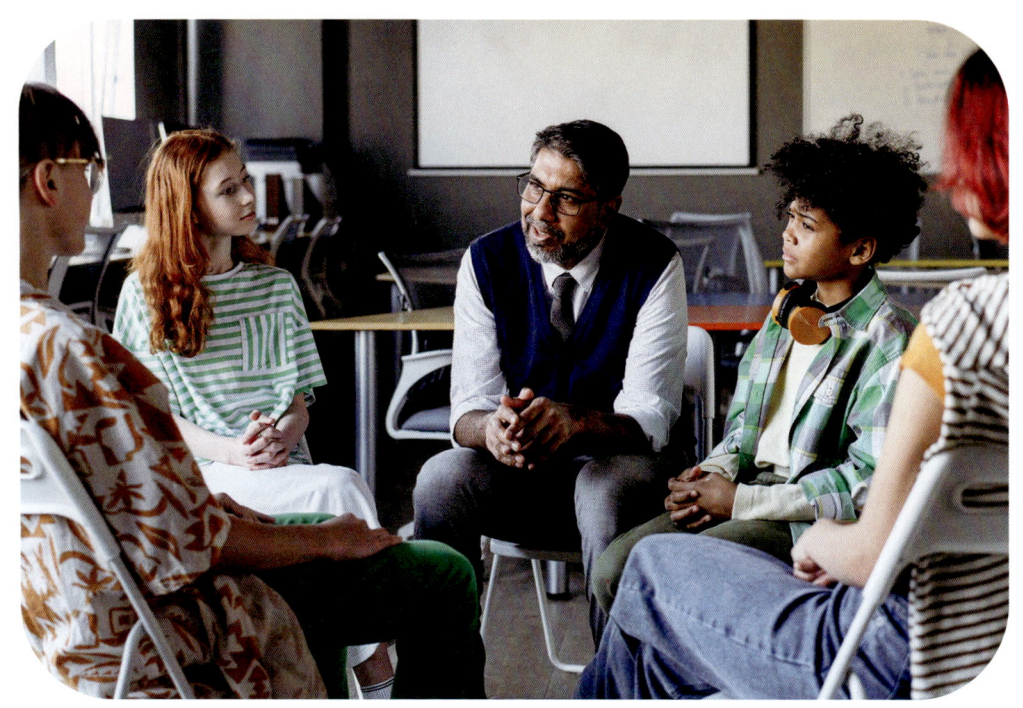

Group therapy can be a safe space for teens to share their struggles and find ways to overcome them.

Psychotherapy can be done in different ways. It may be done one-on-one. This gives someone more personalized care. Therapy may happen with family members. Family therapy is helpful when family issues contribute to depression. Some therapy is done in a group. Group therapy allows people to talk to others with similar struggles. It can help them learn from one another. It may also help teens with depression feel less alone.

Psychotherapy can be done on its own. It can also be done alongside taking medication. Health-care providers may prescribe an **antidepressant** medication.

Selective serotonin reuptake inhibitors, also called SSRIs, are the most common type of antidepressant prescribed to people with depression.

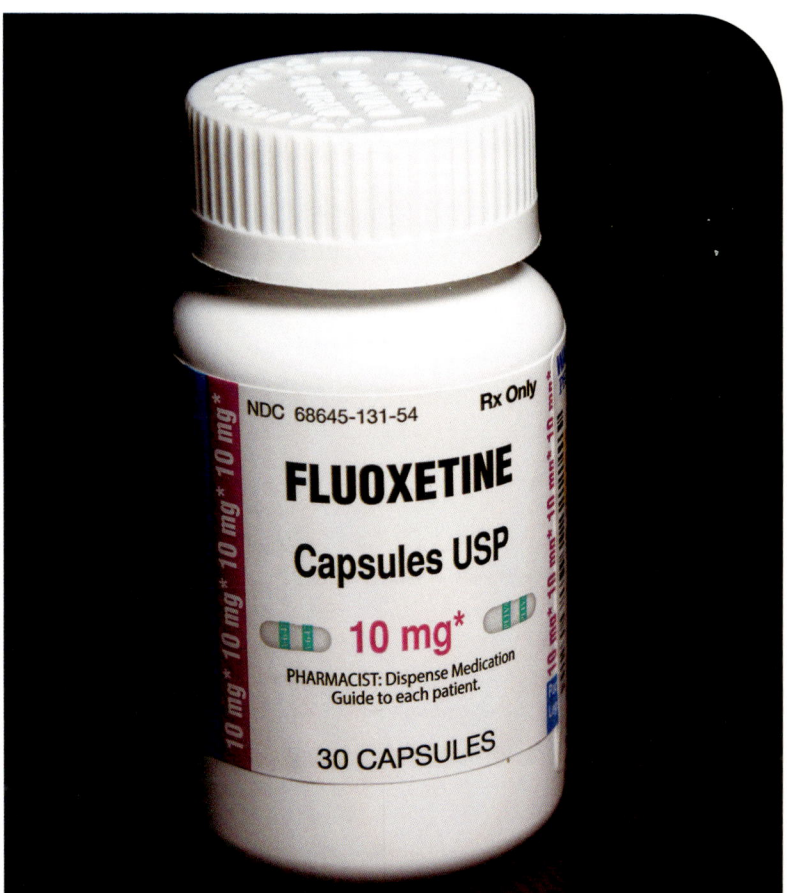

These medicines affect chemicals in the brain that may contribute to the illness.

Jack Bliss developed depression as a teenager. She talked about her struggles. "Everything became painful," she said. "I hated school and dealing with teachers and other students. I hated being at home and

Lifestyle changes, such as exercising regularly, can help treat some people's depression.

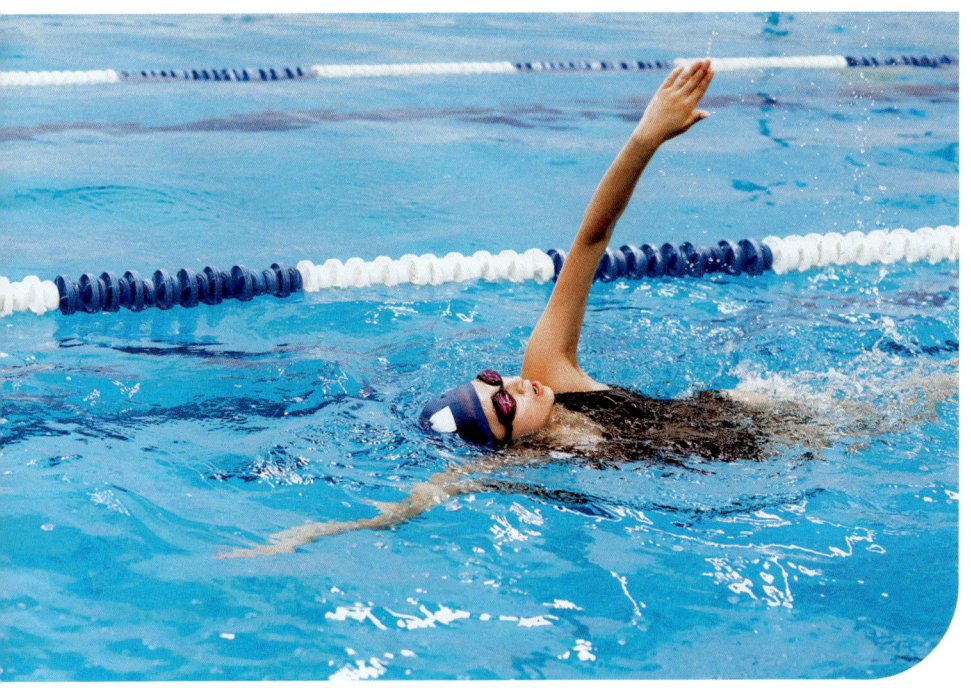

dealing with my family . . . I was constantly putting myself down and thinking about how terrible everything was."[8]

Jack felt overwhelmed by her symptoms. Her recovery began when she told her parents about her mental health struggles. They found Jack a therapist. The therapist helped her deal with her negative thoughts in a better way. Jack also attended group therapy. It was for teens with similar issues. It made her feel less alone.

Jack also saw a **psychiatrist**. They helped her find the right medication. Jack tried a few medicines. She eventually found one that worked for her depression. She continued to meet with a therapist weekly. And over time, she began to feel better.

MEDICATIONS

Finding the right type and dose of medicine can take time. A certain drug or dose may work differently in each person. It may take about 4 to 8 weeks for a medication to take full effect.

Antidepressant medications have possible side effects. Health-care providers watch for certain side effects and help teens manage them. Some teens may need to stop taking an antidepressant. Health-care providers can walk teens through how to safely stop a medication. Quitting suddenly may cause depression to worsen.

HOSPITAL TREATMENT

Some teens have severe depression. They may be in danger of hurting themselves.

In these cases, teens might receive treatment in a hospital. Or they may go to an outpatient program. A hospital stay can keep someone safe and calm while they focus on their treatment. Treatment programs provide support while teens work on their symptoms.

The Suicide Prevention and Counseling Center in Los Angeles, California, provides mental health support for people who have attempted suicide.

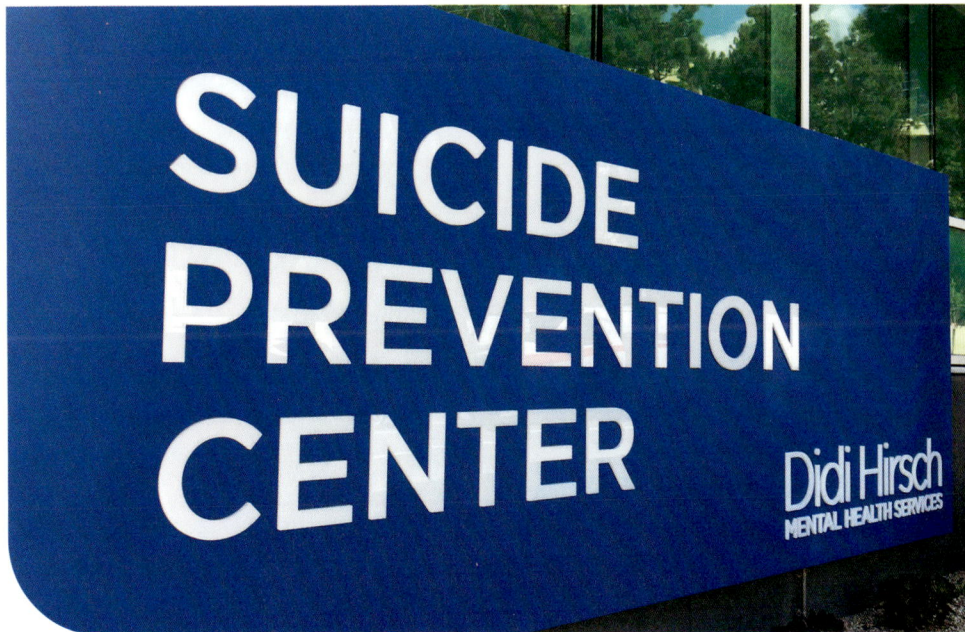

Courtney was 12 years old when she began struggling with depression. She received treatment at a hospital. It helped her on her journey toward getting better. Courtney shared her story to help others. Her advice for teens dealing with depression was to get help. She said it wasn't easy to do. But her treatment helped her get back on track.

MENTAL HEALTH MAINTENANCE

Depression can get better with treatment. But there is no guaranteed way to prevent depression from coming back. Certain factors and experiences may cause another depressive episode. This is why it is important for teens to look after their mental health. Engaging in positive and healthy

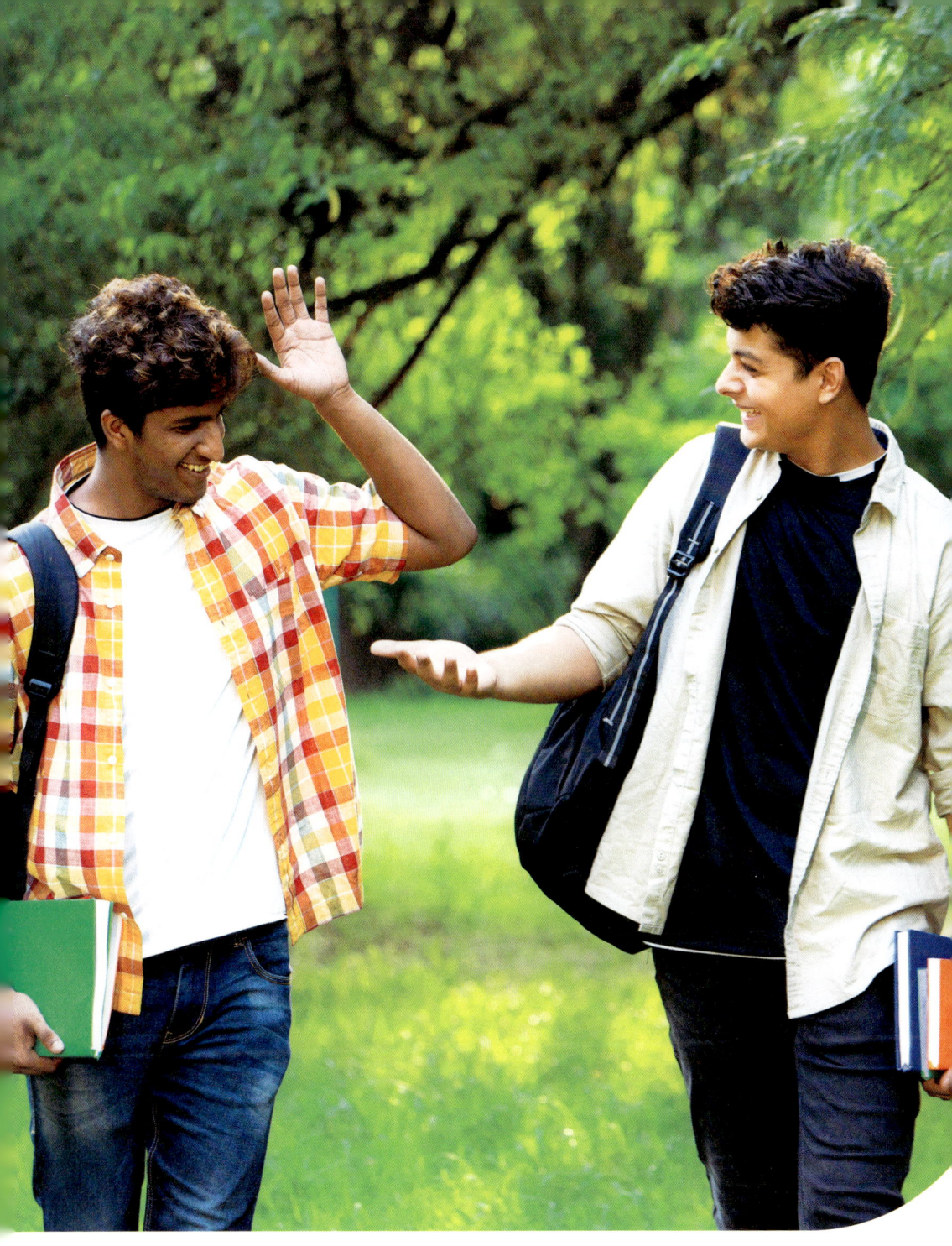

Having a trusted support system can help teens with depression stick to their treatment plan.

actions can help teens better deal with their depression.

Teens can take several steps to decrease the risk of their depression returning. One step is to stick to their treatment plan. Some teens may need to go to therapy longer. Taking medications as prescribed is also important. This is true even if someone feels better.

Taking care of one's physical health can also help manage symptoms. This includes getting regular exercise, eating healthy foods, and getting enough sleep. People with depression should avoid alcohol and drugs. These substances can make treating depression more difficult.

Teens with depression should reach out to friends and family for support.

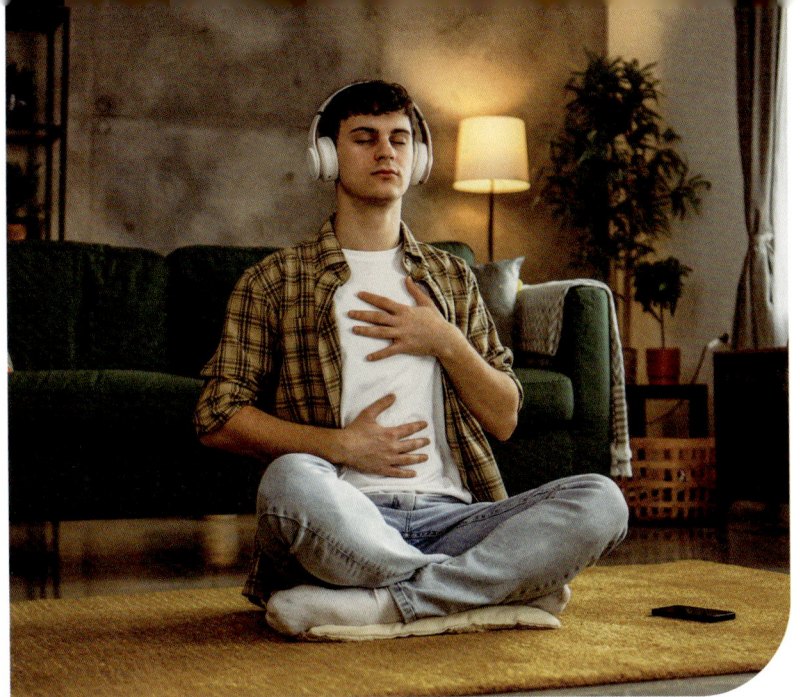

Meditation can help some people better manage their depression.

Feeling connected is important for mental health. In-person socializing is necessary. But technology can play a role too. Online resources can help teens learn more about depression. Therapy sessions can also be done virtually. Teens may use social media to connect to others with similar mental health problems.

Teens can support their mental health by staying active. They can also help themselves by structuring their time. Taking part in enjoyable activities helps people focus on positive emotions. It could mean playing a sport. Or it could be hanging out with friends. Keeping a regular routine can also help lift someone's mood.

Journaling can be a healthy way for teens to lower their stress levels and improve their depression symptoms.

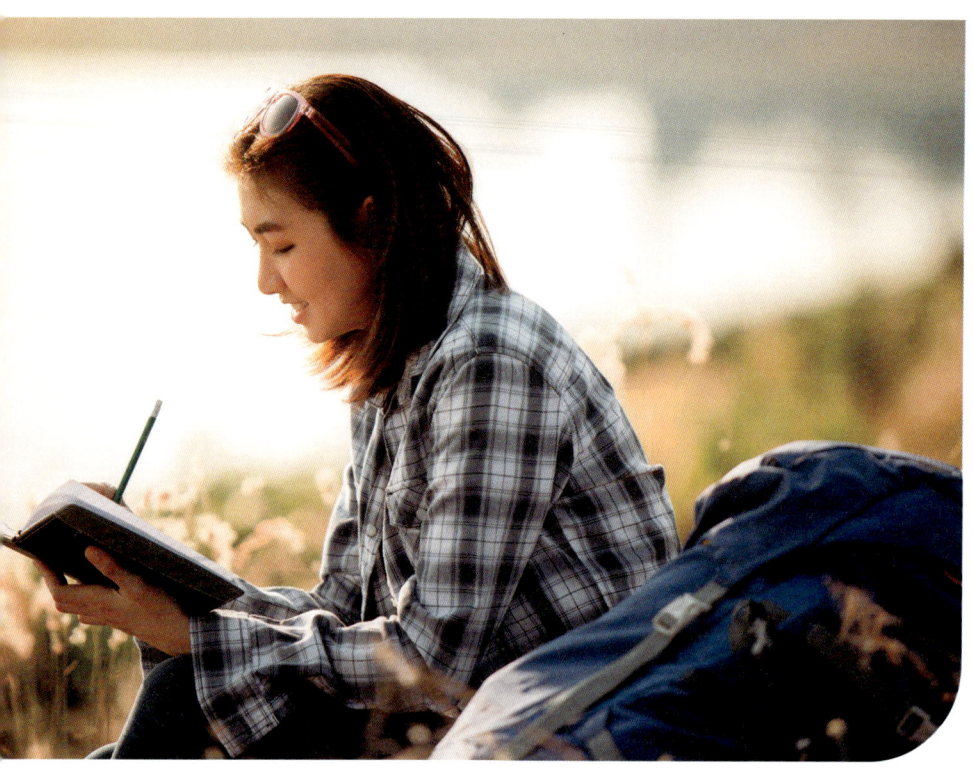

Finally, teens can work to control the stress in their lives. Having reasonable goals and expectations can reduce stress. Some teens also benefit from learning relaxation or **mindfulness** techniques. Mindfulness involves paying attention to the present moment. It can be practiced through meditation. Or it can be done during daily activities. Research shows that mindfulness may help reduce depression.

IT GETS BETTER

Treatment and support have helped many people with their depression. Sam's treatment helped her manage her depression. She went on to college. She studied psychology. Her goal

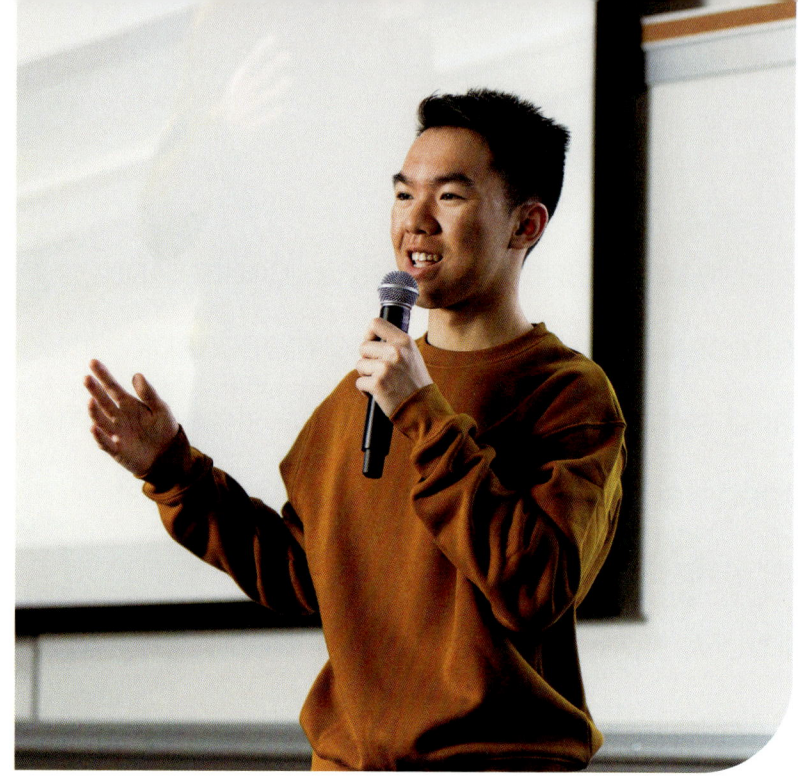

Talking openly about mental health can help lower the negativity surrounding it.

was to help other kids with mental health challenges.

Sam talked about her depression with other young people. She also shared advice. Sam learned that it takes strength to ask for help. Treatment also takes time and effort. But people should realize they are not alone. "There are many more people than you can imagine who have been down the same road and are now living healthy and happy lives," Sam said.[9]

Depression is a serious mood disorder. It affects the lives of millions of teens. But there is always hope. By recognizing the signs, seeking support, and getting treatment, people can overcome depression.

Although many teens have depression, no one has to deal with it alone.

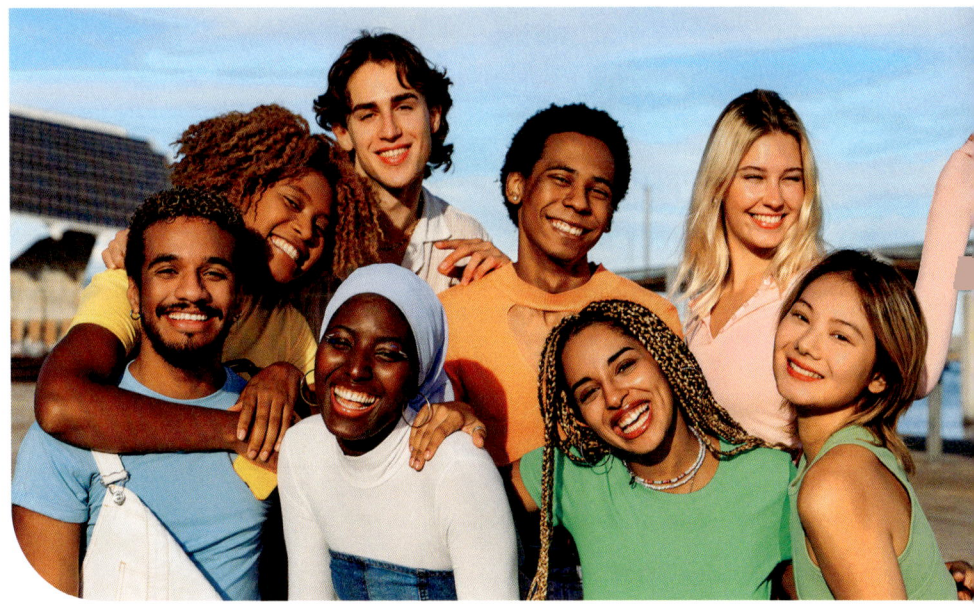

GLOSSARY

antidepressant

a prescription medicine used to treat depression and other mental illnesses

chronic

something that persists for a long time, such as an illness

cope

to manage negative thoughts and feelings to help deal with difficult life situations

diagnosed

identified as the cause of symptoms by a medical professional

inherited

describing things such as traits or illnesses that are passed on from one generation to the next

mindfulness

a state of non-judgmental awareness of the present moment

psychiatrist

a doctor who treats mental health issues

self-esteem

the opinion one has of oneself

SOURCE NOTES

INTRODUCTION: SAM'S STORY

1. Quoted in "Sam's Story," *Franciscan Children's*, n.d. https://franciscanchildrens.org.

CHAPTER ONE: WHAT IS DEPRESSION?

2. Quoted in "What Are Signs of Depression in Teens?" *Scripps*, September 19, 2024. www.scripps.org.

3. Quoted in Mallika Marshall, "How a Mindfulness App May Help Teens Struggling with Depression," *CBS News*, May 17, 2024. www.cbsnews.com.

4. Quoted in Ayesha Rascoe, "The Kids Are Not All Right. The CDC Finds Mental Health Among Teens Has Declined," *NPR*, April 24, 2022. www.npr.org.

CHAPTER TWO: THE IMPACTS OF DEPRESSION

5. Quoted in "Teens Are Talking About Mental Health," *NIH MedlinePlus Magazine*, May 16, 2023. https://magazine.medlineplus.gov.

6. Quoted in "Jordan Burnham Turns Suicide Attempt into Years of Advocacy as Teens Face Epidemic of Depression," *CBS News*, May 19, 2022. www.cbsnews.com.

7. Quoted in "Jordan," *Minding Your Mind*, n.d. https://mindingyourmind.org.

CHAPTER THREE: TREATMENT AND SUPPORT

8. Jack Bliss, "Holding On: A Story About Teen Depression," *CCGC*, n.d. www.ccgcinc.org.

9. Quoted in Franciscan Children's, "A Survivor's Story: 7 Things I Learned from Teen Depression," *Boston Magazine*, n.d. www.bostonmagazine.com.

FOR FURTHER RESEARCH

BOOKS

Hey Gee, *My Life Beyond Depression: A Mayo Clinic Patient Story*. Mayo Clinic Press Kids, 2023.

Mental Health America, *Where to Start: A Survival Guide to Anxiety, Depression, and Other Mental Health Challenges*. Rocky Pond Books, 2023.

Susan Wroble, *Living with Depression*. BrightPoint Press, 2024.

INTERNET SOURCES

"Debunking Myths of Teen Depression," *Johns Hopkins Medicine*, n.d. www.hopkinsmedicine.org.

"Protecting the Nation's Mental Health," *Centers for Disease Control and Prevention*, August 8, 2024. www.cdc.gov.

Melinda Smith, Lawrence Robinson, and Jeanne Segal, "Dealing with Teen Depression," *HelpGuide.org*, August 21, 2024. www.helpguide.org.

WEBSITES

National Alliance on Mental Illness
www.nami.org

The National Alliance on Mental Illness is a nonprofit organization that provides advocacy, education, and public awareness around mental illness. This site offers guidance for people looking for mental health support.

National Institute of Mental Health
www.nimh.nih.gov

The National Institute of Mental Health is a government agency that does research to help understand, treat, and prevent mental illness. This site features information on a variety of mental illnesses, including depression.

Substance Abuse and Mental Health Services Administration
www.samhsa.gov

The Substance Abuse and Mental Health Services Administration is a branch of the US Department of Health and Human Services. It works to reduce the effects of substance abuse and mental illnesses on communities.

INDEX

988 lifeline, 39

American Indian teens, 22, 36

Bliss, Jack, 46–47
bullying, 25
Burnham, Jordan, 36

coping, 8, 10, 31, 33, 43
COVID-19 pandemic, 21–22

depression rates, 18, 22–23, 26
discrimination, 24
disorders, 12, 27, 57

Ethier, Kathleen, 20

factors, 19–20, 24–27, 50

hospital treatment, 48–50
hotlines, 39

isolation, 17, 21

LGBTQ+ teens, 22, 26, 36

managing depression, 50–55
medications, 42–43, 45–48, 52
mental health professionals, 9, 39, 40–43, 45, 47–48
mindfulness, 55
mood changes, 12–15, 17

Native Alaskan teens, 22, 36
negative thoughts, 8, 10, 16–17, 31, 33–35, 43, 47

physical symptoms, 18
programs, 9–10, 49
puberty, 26–27

relationships, 27, 31
resources, 39, 53

school, 21, 26–27, 28–32, 34, 46
self-harm, 8–9, 18, 33–35
signs, 14–16, 37–38, 57
social media, 19–20, 53
stress, 20, 22, 24, 31, 55
substance abuse, 18, 27, 31–32, 52
suicide, 8, 16, 18, 26, 34–39
support, 10, 26, 39, 40, 49, 52–53, 55, 57
symptoms, 15–18, 22, 31, 39, 42, 47, 49, 52

therapy, 42–45, 47, 52–53
treatment access, 42

violence, 20, 24–25

Whitehead, Avary, 16

IMAGE CREDITS

Cover: © Joko P./Shutterstock Images
5: © Monkey Business Images/Shutterstock Images
7: © PeopleImages.com-Yuri A./Shutterstock Images
8: © Vladimir Vladimirov/iStockphoto
9: © Monkey Business Images/Shutterstock Images
11: © New Africa/Shutterstock Images
13: © DimaBerlin/Shutterstock Images
14: © Pics Five/Shutterstock Images
17: © antoniodiaz/Shutterstock Images
21: © S K Tu Mai/Shutterstock Images
23: © Red Line Editorial
25: © Vitchanan Photography/Shutterstock Images
26: © Yta23/Shutterstock Images
29: © Recvisual/iStockphoto
30: © Victor FlowerFly/Shutterstock Images
32: © New Africa/Shutterstock Images
34: © fizkes/Shutterstock Images
37: © ThePalmer/iStockphoto
38: © GagliardiPhotography/Shutterstock Images
41: © Drazen Zigic/iStockphoto
44: © AnnaStills/Shutterstock Images
45: © Wild As Light/Shutterstock Images
46: © Marcos Castillo/Shutterstock Images
49: © Alex Millauer/Shutterstock Images
51: © Master of Stocks/Shutterstock Images
53: © Miljan Zivkovic/Shutterstock Images
54: © AnemStyle/Shutterstock Images
56: © foto-lite/Shutterstock Images
57: © alvarog1970/Shutterstock Images

ABOUT THE AUTHOR

Mary Bates, PhD, is a freelance science writer and author who lives in Rhode Island. She specializes in writing about the brains and behavior of humans and other animals for curious audiences of all ages. She has authored several nonfiction books for young people, including titles on malaria, climate change, and superstitions. When she's not writing, Mary enjoys being in nature, reading, making science crafts, and spending time with her two cats.